George Turner

General View of the Agriculture of the County of Gloucester

With Observations on the Means of Its Improvement

George Turner

General View of the Agriculture of the County of Gloucester With Observations on the Means of Its Improvement

ISBN/EAN: 9783337713690

Printed in Europe, USA, Canada, Australia, Japan

Cover: Foto ©ninafisch / pixelio.de

More available books at **www.hansebooks.com**

GENERAL VIEW

OF THE

AGRICULTURE

OF THE COUNTY OF

GLOUCESTER,

WITH OBSERVATIONS ON THE MEANS OF ITS IMPROVEMENT.

BY

GEORGE TURNER, OF DOWDESWELL.

DRAWN UP FOR THE CONSIDERATION OF THE BOARD OF AGRICULTURE
AND INTERNAL IMPROVEMENT.

LONDON:

PRINTED BY J. SMEETON.

M.DCC.XCIV.

TO THE READER.

*I*T *is requested, that this paper, may be returned to the Board of Agriculture, at its Office in London, with any additional remarks and observations, which may occur on the perusal,* written on the Margin, *as soon as may be convenient.*

It is hardly necessary to add, that the Board does not consider itself responsible for any fact or observation contained in this Report, which at present, is printed and circulated, for the purpose merely of procuring farther information respecting the Husbandry of this district, and of enabling every one, to contribute his mite, to the improvement of the country.

The Board has adopted the same plan, in regard to all the other counties in the united kingdom; and will be happy to give every assistance in its power, to any person, who may be desirous of improving his breed of cattle, sheep, &c. or of trying any useful experiment in husbandry.

London, 1794.

GLOUCESTERSHIRE.

THE county of Gloucester, is bounded on the west by Herefordshire and Monmouthshire, on the north by Worcestershire, on the east by Warwickshire and Oxfordshire, and on the south by Wiltshire and Somersetshire. It contains, according to Bowen's map, about 800,000 acres of land. ·

In describing the agricultural state of the county, it will be necessary to notice separately, the districts differing in soil and management. I begin with the

COTSWOLD HILLS.

The Soil—is various; the greater part, what is here termed " stone brash," a loam intermixed with stones, on a subsoil of calcareous rubble or rock: the average depth of ploughing not much exceeding four inches: there is however some quantity of stiff sour land interspersed on these hills, many farms and one or two whole parishes are chiefly of that nature. Near Fairford and Cirencester the soil is richer and deeper; particularly about the former a deep sandy loam prevails, producing great crops in a favourable time, but apt to burn and parch up in dry seasons; at which times they likewise labour under great inconveniencies for want of water, with which the greater part of these hills is abundantly supplied.

Climate. The Cotswold hills, are milder than could be supposed, from their heighth and deficiency of shelter.
The

The harvest, this last season, was begun in many places, the first week in August, and pretty generally by the second. There is however a difference of from one to three weeks, in the ripening of corn, in the different parts of the district under survey, which cannot be accounted for by management, or any outward circumstances.

The Properties are mostly large, and the occupations likewise; there are however some exceptions in both; but it is the opinion of experienced men, that farms of from 200 to 500 acres, can be managed with much greater advantage to the farmer and the public, than smaller ones.

In the vallies, and where the land is of a sufficient staple for permanent meadow and pasture, it is mostly in that state. Sheep and cow downs are likewise frequently met with; but the quantity of land thus employed, bears but a small proportion, to that which is occasionally under the plough; some few parishes on the sides of the hills however, are an exception to this rule, in which perhaps half the land is meadow and pasture, worth from 20 to 30s. per acre. In these situations, dairying is mostly followed, in preference to grazing; the sort of cows chiefly Gloucestershire, frequently crossed and improved from other breeds. Most farmers dairy a little for home consumption; and though the nature of the soil, renders sheep the live stock chiefly to be attended to, yet a sufficient quantity of cattle, generally are, and always ought to be, intermixed with them to improve the pastures, and make the most of the keep; of these not so many are bred as formerly, Gloucester market weekly affording great choice from Herefordshire, Wales and Somersetshire; of these, the Glamorgan and Somerset appear most eligible as working cattle for the hills, being active in harness, and when turned off, feeding in less time than the larger breed of Herefordshire. In stall-feeding, hay,

hay, chaff, barleymeal, oats and bran* are the articles
of food chiefly used. The smaller Welch breeds of cattle
where grazing is the only object, are frequently bought
in in winter or early in spring, and fatted in the course
of the summer, so as to go off between Michaelmas and
Christmas with little or no hay, which in a country
where it is so scarce and valuable, is a material object.

The native *sheep* of these hills in their unimproved state,
was a small light carcassed, polled animal, bearing in the
memory of an experienced agriculturist now living, a
fleece of fine wool of about 3 lb. weight, but lighter and
finer before that period. They were cotted in former
times, but that practice has not been in use since the
remembrance of the person alluded to, from which
circumstances it is very propable that the assertions of
ancient authors, that the Spaniards procured their breed
of fine woolled sheep from the Cotswold Hills, are founded
in fact, though contradicted by some modern writers.
Since that time the inclosures and better management
taking place, and good rams being procured from Warwickshire and other counties, the Cotswold sheep have
considerably improved in weight of carcass and quantity
of wool, which, though coarser than formerly, is in
very great esteem as combing wool, being of a good length
and very mellow quality. The fashionable Leicestershire
sheep have been occasionally introduced into this district,
and, for a cross or two when chosen with judgement,

* If a mill could be invented to grind wheat, either by the wind or with a
horse, cheap and durable, it would enable the farmer by mealing his own grain,
to obtain a quantity of excellent food for his fatting stock, to the great enrich-
ment of the land. The great objection to the steel mills hitherto invented,
is, that the corn must be in the very best order, otherwise it clogs and will not
grind properly. To make a machine of this sort complete and generally useful,
there must probably be some ingenious contrivance annexed to dry and harden
the corn if necessary.

have

have been found to improve the breed in shape and dispo-
sition to fatten, but where persisted in, they have greatly
reduced the carcass in size, and considerably lessened the
wool in quality and quantity: nor is this reduction in
size recompenced by their requiring less food, or fattening
quicker than the other breeds, qualities which have been
so strongly insisted on, and on which the merit of the
breed has been chiefly founded; on the contrary, experienced graziers in this district who have paid particular
attention to them, are convinced, that they require full
as much time and room as the larger native breed.   I say
nothing of the comparative value of the carcasses to the
butcher, nor of the estimation the meat of the different
breeds is held in by the consumer; the most satisfactory
intelligence on these heads may be obtained in Smithfield
Market.

In the common practice of the district the wether sheep
are fatted off from two to three years old. The average
weight of carcasses, ewe 22 lb. wether 26 lb. per quarter;
fleeces on an average of the whole flock run four to the tod
of 28 lb.   Wool sold this season from 14s. to 24s.
per tod. I understood at this time it is not worth more
than 18s.

Wether sheep, by keeping them another year, are
frequently brought to weigh from 40 to 50lb. the quarter.

Probably no part of the kingdom has been more improved
within the last forty years, than the Cotswold Hills.   The
first inclosures are about that standing; but the greater
part are of a later date.   Three parishes are now inclosing;
and out of about thirteen, which still remain in the common field state, two I understand are taking the requisite
measures for an inclosure; the advantages are great, rent
more than doubled, the produce of every kind proportion-
ably increased.   In the open field state, a crop and fallow
was the usual course.   What is here called the " seven-
field husbandry" now generally obtains; that is, about
                                    a seventh

a seventh part sainfoin, and the remainder under the following routine; turnips, barley, seeds two years, wheat, oats. A part of the wheat stubble is sometimes sowed with peas, but generally more with a view to home consumption than for sale, that crop being very precarious, if often repeated. Vetches are likewise frequently, though not so often as they should be, substituted for the oat crop, to be eaten on the land with sheep, or mowed for horses and other stock. The management of the crops requires to be more particularly described.

Sainfoin.—This district stands one of the first in the cultivation of this excellent grass; the usual management has been to sow it with barley, after turnips, three bushels per acre, to which is generally added about five pounds of trefoil, which generally improves the first year's produce, and by occupying the soil, prevents the weeds from getting a-head till the sainfoin has established its roots. There are some very superior managers, however, who having been induced from an accidental occurrence to think a different procedure would be more advantageous, tried it with so much success, that they have constantly adhered to it since. The method alluded to, is to sow it on land exhausted by repeated cropping and full of couch grass, the sainfoin rooting so deep, does not draw its nourishment like corn, from the surface soil, and therefore is not injured by its impoverished state, whilst its greatest enemy, the black bent, is effectually kept under by the couch grass. In this practice it is likewise sown with barley, and very thin, not more than a bushel per acre, it having been noticed by the same attentive observers, that, when sown thin, the roots are larger and more vigorous, and in two or three years get full possession of the land, producing greater crops, and lasting longer than the thicker planted. There are other practitioners who object to thin sowing, observing that the hay being chiefly wanted for

sheep,

sheep, although it may produce as much or more in quantity, the stems are much larger and not so palatable to that animal, occasioning great waste in the consumption. It must likewise be observed, that the method of sowing it on foul exhausted land, having been tried in the neighbourhood of Gusting, on a less genial soil, has in two instances that have come to my knowledge, failed; it might therefore be advisable, when the culture is new, to make small experiments first. In the neighbourhood of Stowe, I am informed, a fourth part of the land is appropriated to this grass; but as it requires a great many years to intervene before land that has once borne it, can be cropped with success, that probably may be found too large a proportion. The duration of sainfoin depends a great deal on the management; mowing it before its full blossom is detrimental, the roots bleeding very much and mildewing; for the same reason seeding of it is accounted beneficial; if wished to last, it should never be fed but in the months of October and November, and then only with cattle, sheep biting too close; the lattermath is, however, excellent food for weaned lambs, and therefore often applied to that purpose. Indeed the farmers in general do not wish it to last longer than seven years; the land being in that time thoroughly rested and fit for corn, whilst other land under the plough wants rest; but if desired, it might, with proper management, last ten or twelve years. The hay, if well made, is, in the fore part of the season, equal to any meadow hay in the district for most purposes. When worn out, so as not to be worth mowing, it is generally pastured a year or two, which thickens the turf, and of course produces more and better ashes, when pared and burnt, in which method it is always broken up.

Turnips—in the usual practice, succeed oats; the stubble is ploughed in autumn or the beginning of winter, in which state it lies till spring seed-time is finished, when,

being

being well dragged, it receives two or more ploughings, if necessary, with sufficient dragging and harrowing between, and allowing as much time as possible between each operation, for the seeds of weeds to vegetate and be destroyed. The dung of the farm yard is chiefly applied to this crop. They are sown from the latter end of May to the beginning of August, and once or twice hoed, according to circumstances. They are eaten off with sheep; always beginning at the lower part of the ground, and working up hill ; plenty of hay is allowed, which in this district is necessary for the health and well-doing of the animal. Turnips, thus expended, greatly enrich the land, and are found of use through the whole course of crops.

Barley—is sown after turnips, on one ploughing, as soon as the peas and oats are got in the ground. Grass seeds are either sown before the last time of the harrows, or after the barley is come up, and before rolling it ; in which case it is usually covered in with a bush hurdle: quantity of seed three bushels ; average produce twenty-four bushels per acre.

Grass seeds—chiefly sown, are from two to six pecks ray grass, and from five to ten pounds trefoil ; likewise a small quantity of broad and white Dutch clover ; but the light land is apt to tire of the broad clover, if often sown in quantity ; and the white Dutch is getting out of repute for sheep feed. In the common practice the seeds are mown for hay the first year, and grazed the following summer, when the land is ploughed up for wheat.

A very valuable sort of *ray grass*, which has been cultivated for twenty years past, by Mr. Peacey, of North Leach, deserves particular mention. Perhaps there is no grass existing more valuable to the stock farmer than this, if properly managed ; it is very early, and affords a great quantity of excellent keep before any other pastures will

carry

carry stocks: a ground of it, hined the preceding Michaelmas, kept eight ewes with their lambs per acre for one month last spring, before any other pasture was ready for them. It is very nourishing, and grateful to all kinds of stock; as may be seen where they have a choice of that and other pastures to run in, the natural pastures will be quite neglected, whilst the ray grass will be pared close to the ground: indeed it requires to be hard stocked; for if suffered to get a-head, it is neither so palatable, nor nourishing; it is equally excellent for hay, if cut just as the ear appears, and before it is fully formed; in the autumn, it likewise affords a great deal of keep. It rather improves with age, and has been found particularly advantageous, in laying land down to permanent pasture. It has not been a general practice, with the farmers on these hills, to raise their ray grass seed; the deficiency of natural pastures, and the large flocks of sheep kept, making the lays valuable, both for hay and pasture; this has occasioned rather a scarcity of seed of late years, and been the means of introducing very inferior sorts from other countries, of which some have proved strictly annual, producing a tolerable crop the first year, but dying away the following winter; whilst that of longer duration has been found very unproductive, particularly, all the latter part of the season. The great loss and injury sustained by these failures, has made the farmers more attentive in their choice of seed, and greatly advanced the price of that which can be relied on; so that Mr. Peacey seeded an unusual quantity last year, to answer the demand which he foresaw he should have for it; it is already engaged at the advanced price of half a guinea per bushel, which price was fixed on it by some gentlemen who had experienced its value, and thought it would not only properly reward the attention which had preserved so valuable a grass, but be the means of making it more generally known, and encouraging the culture of it, to the exclusion

of

of all the inferior sorts. Mr. Peacey has likewise cultivated the orchis grass, a broad-leaved grass, that springs
directly after the scythe, in mowing grounds; he finds this
very useful on barren land, that will bear no other grass.
A bank of this description, adjoining his downs, is covered with the orchis grass, and from the stock lying on it,
and paring it down, it seems very palatable to them.

Wheat.—The method of sowing this grain in the district
under notice, is rather singular. The land is ploughed from
two to six weeks before sowing, as circumstances permit;
if it gets quite grassy, it is thought better. The first rain
that falls in August in sufficient quantity to thoroughly
soak the land, begins the seed time; from thence to the
middle of September is thought the best time, The seed is
dragged in with heavy drags, working the land till the
furrows are well broke, but rather wishing to leave it rough
than otherwise; if frequent showers fall during the dragging in, so as just to allow the drags to work, it is thought
better by most people. Experienced men say, that our land
being naturally too light for wheat, is by these means,
rendered more suitable to it, at the same time that weeds
are very much checked, which is a very material object,
where the corn is so long on the ground. I have seen
adjoining lands, the previous management of which had
been exactly similar, the one part sown wet, produced a
very good crop for the country, and quite clean; the other,
sown dry, was not half so good, and devoured with filth.
This method is practised on the dry sound loams, of which
the district chiefly consists; on the heavier soils, attention is paid to the state in which they work best. the stiff
sour land is frequently fallowed and dunged for wheat,
over which broad clover is often harrowed in; in spring,
after lying one or two years, it is broke up for wheat, followed by oats; or sometimes oats are sown on the lay,
according to the state of the land. Turnips are sometimes

times sown on this sort of land, but, perhaps, had better
be omitted; the poaching, in eating off, possibly doing
more injury, than the teeth of the sheep recompences,
rendering it unfit for any crop but oats, and probably
injuring them. Wheat, clover, and oats, seem to be
the crops best adapted to these soils. Cabbages are not
known here, in field culture, and probably these kinds
of soils would require more dung, than the situation could
command to cultivate that plant to any advantage. It may
be right to notice, in this place, an error of Marshall's,
in his Rural Economy of Gloucestershire, vol. 2, page 33.
He represents the Cotswold farmers as " wishing to plough
for every crop, when the soil is wet, and working even
their fallows, when they are moist." This mistake ori-
ginated, no doubt, from the account given him of the
wheat process, as just related. The fact is, the farmers
here are as desirous of working their fallows in dry weather, and find the same good consequences resulting from
it, as in other districts. Attention is likewise paid to
sowing the barley in dry weather. The old adage respecting pease, " if you sow in a flood, they will come up in a
wood," seems verified on this soil; as for oats, their har-
diness requires no particular nicety. Such an error is very
excusable in an account which is only given as an excur-
sion. Mr. Marshall's account of this county contains
much valuable information, and has greatly shortened
mine.

Oats.—The wheat stubble is mowed, if worth it, or
otherwise harrowed, when it becomes brittle enough to
break off, and casted to the fold-yard; and the land
ploughed as soon as leisure and the weather will permit,
for Oats, which are harrowed in as soon as the land will
work, in February, about four bushels per acre, average
produce 24 bushels.

Peas

Peas are sown as early as possible in spring, the sort mostly in use is the early Burbage; they are generally ploughed in under furrow, about five bushels per acre, average produce twenty-four bushels.

Winter Vetches are, in the practice of a few individuals, sown in quantity to eat off with store sheep; they are usually sown after wheat, as soon after harvest as opportunity allows. The sheep are put on them the latter end of May, or beginning of June. They are commonly hurdled off in the same manner as turnips; but if a bulky crop, the better way is to give them through rack hurdles, which are made the same as the common five railed ones, only leaving the middle rail out, and nailing spars across at proper distances, to admit the sheep to put their heads through. A swarth of vetches being mown across the lands, a sufficient number of these hurdles, allowing one to five sheep, are set close to it; at noon the shepherd mows another swarth, and throws it to the hurdles, and the same at night; next morning, a swarth being first mowed, the hurdles are again set; thus moving them once in twenty-four hours; by this trifling additional trouble, the vetches are clean eaten off, and the land equally benefitted. As fast as the lands are cleared, they are ploughed, and sown with turnips, in which way good crops are often obtained in kind seasons, on land cleared in tolerable time, but it cannot be depended on for the main crop. When a succession is wanted, spring vetches are sometimes sowed; but at the time they are sown, labour is more valuable, and besides, they are not so much to be depended on.

Manures are chiefly those of the fold-yard. The wheat stubbles are frequently mown or raked for litter, and cattle kept in sufficient quantity to eat the straw, but this is not always the case; large heaps of straw are seen in some parts of the district, rotting at the barn doors, for

want

want of cattle to eat and tread it into dung, and this generally for want of a sufficiency of pasture to support the stock in summer; but surely, the keeping more land down to grass, or raising some sort of vegetable food for such stock, would be ultimately attended with increase of produce and profit to the farmer, and advantage to the public. The formation of the fold yards, so as to prevent the rain water from washing the dung heaps, as well as preserving the liquid part of manure, is not at all attended to, though so much deserving of attention; on the contrary, from the sloping situations of many of the fold-yards, it might be imagined, that the prime object in laying them out, was to diminish the value of the dung heaps as much as possible. Ashes from burnt turf, or grassy stubbles, are very beneficial, and such land is usually broken up in that way. Lime is too expensive for manure; nor from two or three experiments that have come under my observation, does it seem worth attention, if that was not the case. Soot has been tried on sainfoin to great advantage, but it is not to be procured in sufficient quantity for any considerable practice. Marl has been formerly used in different parts of the district; a pit has been opened of late years in the neighbourhood of Northleach, to the great improvement of some adjoining grass grounds. Folding sheep is very little practised or approved of. The observations in the Annals of Agriculture on that practice, are well deserving of attention.

Watering meadows, has long been practised in this district; there is, probably, no considerable quantity of land capable of that improvement, without interfering with the mills, where it is not done.

Implements of husbandry—The waggon of this district is described by Mr. Marshall, and by him allowed to be the best in the kingdom for husbandry uses. The testimony of Mr. Drake, given to the Worcestershire surveyor, tends

to

to confirm that idea. The carts are very good for hauling
out dung, but not so well calculated for road work and
other uses. The ploughs are long in the beam, with one
wheel; they are rather improved in their construction of
late. Four horses or four or five oxen the most usual
draught; in spring seed time and s'irring fallows, generally
less. It is most probable ploughs might be invented to
do the work as well with less strength; but the land in
general being a tenacious loam, full of stones, is more
tiresome to the cattle, and requires more strength than
would seem necessary on a superficial view.

Horses and Oxen are both used, the latter in harness, and
getting ground, but not so much as they ought. One team
of horses is necessary for carrying out corn, on our rough
and hilly roads, but where more than one team is kept,
oxen certainly are in every respect the most eligible.
Where the farms are large or not handy to the homestall, a
wooden house, fixed on a sledge, is used to hold the ox
harness, which being drawn to the ground where the
beasts are pastured, and as convenient as can be to their
work, saves a great deal of time and unnecessary' tra-
velling. The same cabbins, if made with sparred bottoms and lids to open on each side, are very useful occasionally to keep fattening calves in.

Farm Houses and Offices in the old inclosures, are frequently unhandy and inadequate to the farms annexed to
them, which, doubtless, arises from the improvements in
husbandry since their building. In the new inclosures,
they are generally speaking very conveniently situated, with
sufficient shed room for cattle and implements. In the
modern improved method of inclosing, it is thought best
to divide the arable part of the farm into seven inclosures
of equal size, being the number required for the most ap-

proved

proved course of crops, allowing two or three smaller patches near home for odd purposes.

The Fences are usually dry stone walls, good quarries of which are generally very handy. Quick hedges are sometimes planted, but the attention and time required to raise them is a great objection. In one or two instances they have been planted within side the walls with great success—it is a pity the practice is not more general.

Population is supposed to have increased on these hills of late years, and it is generally believed that inclosures by finding more employment, tends very much to promote at least, useful population. The small pox frequently makes great ravages in the country—it is a pity a general inoculation did not take place every five or six years, which would be a great saving in expence to the different parishes, as well as the preserving many useful lives.

Prices of Labour are considerably increased; from 12d. to 14d. a day in winter; 18d. to 20d. haymaking; harvest 2s; beer or an allowance in malt in some places, is gaining ground, and as much as possible, is done by the great. Women from 6d. to 8d. and 9d. in haymaking; in harvest 12d. Hours of work from six to six, when day-light permits; late hours in haymaking, and harvest generally recompenced with beer, &c.

The Value of Draining has been long understood and practised in this district, old drains of wood and stone being frequently met with in making new ones. A great deal has been done of late years; there is still much to do; but some of the stiff sour land that most wants it, is of so retentive a nature, that the drains will not draw to the least distance. Probably Mr. Elkington's method, as mentioned in the Annals of Agriculture, Vol. 16, page 544,

544, might be beneficial. The chief material is stone, the methods of doing it varies, but have nothing new from those described in different parts of the Annals. Probably digging the trenches sufficiently deep and filling with stone, where it is handy, will be found the most cheap and lasting method. In doing this the largest stone should be put in first, and the surface levelled with smaller ones, sprinkling a little straw on the top, to prevent the loose mould from getting between; or for want of that, the grassy sides of the sods turned down will answer the same purpose.

Paring and Burning is very much practised and approved; old sainfoin lays and all turf of a sufficient texture are usually broke up in that way. Turnips are often the first crop; and from the freshness of the land, and the good effects of the ashes, a large crop is generally obtained. But as the time is too short to get the land in proper tilth for the succeeding crops of barley, seeds, &c. it is thought a better method to sow wheat first, on one ploughing; after which, the ashes being still fresh in the ground, a crop of turnips may be as safely relied on, and there is plenty of time to get the land in compleat tilth. Grassy wheat stubbles, that will produce a tolerable quantity of ashes, are frequently pared and burnt for turnips with great success. .In short whenever followed with the turnip and clover husbandry, its good effects are indisputable; but like every other practice, it is liable to abuse in the hands of designing men, who have sometimes made use of it to force repeated crops of corn, 'till the soil has been compleatly worn out and rendered incapable of any useful production*.

* Down Ampney and its neighbourhood, the part of this county that borders on Wiltshire, is the only place in which I have met with any objections to this management; the soil here consists of stiff clays and gravels; on the clays they do not think it answers, but approve of it on the gravels.

Coppices

Coppices are very much wanted in this district. Ash thrives remarkably well on this soil, and is very useful for hurdles and gates, as well as for fuel, which is a very scarce article; the coppices we have are chiefly composed of this wood, which is fetched from a great distance for coopers, and other uses; and has greatly risen in price, as well as got scarcer of late years, so as to cause serious apprehensions in some parts of the district, of great inconveniencies for want of a sufficient supply of this useful article. It is a great pity that every estate had not a sufficient quantity planted to supply the tenantry and labourers dependant on it. Odd corners, and sour patches, of little use under the plough, might be very profitably applied to this purpose; in boggy ground, too wet for the ash, the alder thrives well, and is very useful for gates, hurdles, and other common purposes. It has been found, that ash will not grow on the tops of the hills, though it thrives very well on the slopes; but there are a great many such situations in this district, which if planted with Scotch firs, beach, or any hardy trees that would grow, would add much to the beauty of the country, as well as greatly improve the soil and climate of the adjoining land, by the shelter they afforded. The chief woodlands are in the parishes of Chedworth, Withington, and Dowdeswell, smaller patches in Guiting and one or two neighbouring parishes; these are looked on as the natural production of the soil, protected and encouraged of late years. They are cut at about 18 years growth, and produce from 30£. to 60£. per acre. There are some coppices consisting chiefly of ash, in the parishes of Wick and Slaughter, that have been planted in modern times; they are first cut at 10 years growth, afterwards generally at about 18 years growth, and produce from 25£. to 60£. per acre. Great attention is here paid to keeping them clean, by hoeing for two or three years after cutting, 'till the young

shoots

shoots are sufficiently strong to smother the weeds. Alder coppices are cut at 12 years growth, and are worth from 15£. to 25£. per acre.

Roads, both public and parochial, are very much improved of late years.

Manufactures—The woollen manufactories supply spinning work to the poor women, in many parts of the district, but the earnings are very low. Some quantity of home spun linen is likewise brought to Stowe and other fairs, for common uses.

Leases—I know of nothing commendable in the leases of the district; a good plain form, equally protecting the interest of landlord and tenant, is much wanting, if possible to be drawn. At present they are chiefly in professional hands, who either content themselves with antiquated copies, or, in order to guard against trifling inconveniencies, cramp the industrious tenant, so as often to prevent improvements to the advantage of himself, his landlord, and the community; whilst, at the same time, they do not prevent the knave and sloven from running into the contrary extreme.

It has already been noticed, that this district has been greatly improved of late years; it is still improving, nor is any spirit of that sort wanting; but it might be greatly assisted by the removal of some of the burthens, that the farming world in general labour under. Among these, the payment of tythes in kind deserve to be mentioned. In the new inclosures, this load has been got rid of by giving up a part of the property in lieu of it. One-fifth of the arable, and one-ninth of the pasture, and in some instances, two-ninths of one, and one-eighth of the other, has been asked, and agreed to. As the impropriator is exonerated from all expences, except inside fences, the

part

part that he takes is more than equal to a fourth of the arable land, even when one-fifth is allowed; but even then the improvements being entirely the proprietors, they have been obliged to acquiesce. The acts of Parliament allow the rectors only to lease for the first twenty-one years, and afterwards the tenants remain tenants at will; in consequence of which, all the lands set apart for the clergy, become, in a great measure, unproductive; as the tenants take from them all they can raise, and set every improvement aside; and therefore they are so far neither beneficial to the clergy, or the nation. But were commissioners appointed to value the tythes of the parishes, and also the landed estates of the clergy, and were they obliged, under that valuation, to grant leases, at the rent then set on them, their estates would be improved, in proportion as other lands; and the tythes being secured to the occupiers, for a term, not exceeding twenty-one years, they could have no objection to the advance to be made on them at the expiration of that term, and the difficulties now existing, would be done away, in so far as respects the occupiers and the nation. The rent to be paid for the land, would be of no consequence in what proportion it was paid; as the only security requisite to the occupiers, is that on laying out their capital they may have from the impropriator an equal term with that they have from their landlords, and to put both on an equal footing. As the law now stands, the burden may be immoderate, and therefore to every person acquainted with the value of money (which the farmers are now, more than formerly) and know how to make calculations, it cannot be expected that they will lay out any considerable sum, when the first 11 per cent. profit, goes to the impropriator, before they can receive any advantage themselves: and, in case of a loss, that loss is augmented by the impropriators taking a tenth part of the capital laid out, as far as it was returned to the occupiers.

Par

Poor Rates are every where increasing. The administration of the poor laws, not only takes a large sum yearly, from the agriculturist, but, in its effects, greatly injures him, by encouraging idleness and profligacy, among the labouring poor. The liberal orders for relief, which an artful tale, and an appearance of poverty and wretchedness, most generally occasioned by sloth and debauchery, has too often obtained, has held out a means of support independent of manual labour and exertion, and quite destroyed that laudable pride, which, a few years ago was often to be observed among the labouring poor, of keeping themselves independent of their parishes ; on the contrary, the most trifling accidents now bring them to the overseers, and from thence to the magistrates, for relief. Real policy, justice, and humanity, require that parish relief should be administered in such a sparing manner, as to convince those liable to be beholden to it, that they must look to their own exertions and industry alone for a comfortable subsistence. If an alteration in the poor laws, which is much to be wished for, does not take place, let it be recommended to all large parishes, to establish workhouses for their paupers, and let small parishes be encouraged to join in doing the same, and suffer no relief to be granted out of them. The good effects of which has been found in many instances in this county, and shortly corroborate what has been advanced above, that profligacy and idleness, more than real want, has brought the poor's tax to such an enormous height.

Ale-Houses are a very great nuisance to the farmer, and the public ; they hold out too great a temptation to the labourer to waste that money in debauchery, which ought to find bread for his family, and greatly assist the idle and wicked servant in corrupting his fellows and making them as bad as himself. The magistrates of this county, have laudably exerted themselves in suppressing houses of this

description

description; there are still too many. Those only ought to be suffered, that are absolutely necessary for the accommodation of travellers.

Chandlers Shops are nearly as great a nuisance in country places, as ale-houses. They retail, in small quantities and at extravagant rates, the worst of commodities; and draw that money out of the pockets of the poor for tea, sugar, butter, and other unnecessary articles, which, if taken to a proper market, and well laid out, would support themselves and families in health and comfort. If a plan could be devised to furnish the poor in their respective parishes with necessary articles, good in quality, and at the lowest market price, I know of nothing that would so effectually relieve them. Here are some neighbouring instances of a saving of 18d. or 2s. a week, for a family of five or six people, in the article of bread only, by their being supplied with flour at the best hand.

Dogs are now so generally kept by working men, as to become a great nuisance; they worry, injure, and sometimes kill the farmer's sheep; and, it is generally allowed, are, from their bad keep, most liable to madness; besides, that there can be no other inducement to the poor man for keeping them, but for the purposes of poaching; which is not only contrary to law, but leads to idle and vicious habits, and generally ends in worse crimes. A tax on dogs might not only prevent this, but likewise reduce the number of useless ones kept by people in a higher station.

THE STROUDWATER HILLS.

The soil on the hills is chiefly light loam; not so tenacious as the Cotswolds, nor so productive; there is likewise some quantity of sour wet land; the climate is nearly similar to the Cotswolds; the properties are various as are

the

the size of the farms. On the hills, strictly speaking, it is supposed, nine-tenths of the land is arable. The approved course of crops, the same as before, noted of the Cotswolds. On the vallies there are large tracts of good meadow land, which is applied both to grazing and the dairy; but mostly, the latter. There is some quantity of land watered, and a great deal more is capable of that improvement: but the mills interfere greatly; for the dairies the cattle are chiefly bred, and are in general good; in grazing, the stock is more generally bought in, and are of various breeds, according to their application, the opinion of the grazier, and the goodness of the land.

Sheep, on the hills, are the chief stock; these are mostly of the horned Wiltshire bred, the fleeces average nine to the tod of 28 lbs. worth this year 26s. 6d. per tod. Average weight, when fat, wether 24 lbs. ewe 22 lbs. per quarter. This breed is liable to a disorder called the Goggles, which sometimes occasions very heavy losses. The only method of prevention is, entirely changing the flock once in eight or ten years. One practitioner, Mr. Hayward, of Baverstone, has been induced, from this circumstance, to try the Cotswold breed, and having, for three or four years past, used rams of that breed, he will very soon entirely get rid of the Wiltshire blood; and, I am inclined to think, will find a great advantage in so doing.

The Rotation of Crops, it has been observed, is similar to that on the Cotswolds. I saw here an application of turnips, quite new to me. Mr. Hayward gives them in quantity to his farm horses, which he finds keeps them very healthy, and induces them to eat the barn chaff, and other dry meat, with a better appetite;—they were, when I saw them, in very good condition, though, I was informed, they had had no corn for half a year past, and were constantly worked. The Cotswold farmer can sel-

dom

dom procure turnips in sufficient quantity for such an application, nor would he chuse to deprive his land of the benefit derived from their being eat on it by sheep, except the crop was very heavy, in which case, perhaps, they might be advantageously thinned a little, for this purpose, or for fattening cattle in stalls. This gentleman, and his neighbour, Mr. Tugwell, cultivate the turnip-rooted cabbage. Mr. Tugwell's crop is very fine; they are transplanted on to ridges, formed by a *bout* of a double mould-board plough, of his own invention; he finds they will not flourish with him, without transplanting. This crop comes to perfection, when the turnips are all spent, and supports a great stock, just in the scarce time of spring, which makes it particularly valuable. Mr. Tugwell has likewise cultivated the Roota baga, which he does not at present approve of, but means to give it farther trial.

This gentleman is the inventor of the two-horse plough, which has been honourably noticed in the Transactions of the Bath Society, and which I understand he is now requested by them to draw up a particular account of. I saw several of them at work in a ground of Mr. Hayward's; they seemed to go very easy to the horses, and made very good work. Mr. D. Hayward informed me that in a trial of ploughing among some neighbours, they ploughed an acre of clover ley, with one of these ploughs, and a single horse in six hours. These ploughs have been tried on the Cotswold Hills; but the persons who tried them never entertained an idea, that the horses could go in them for eight or nine hours, without baiting, as is practised here; and the introduction of the Norfolk custom of baiting at noon and working later in the evening, though by no means a bad one, yet being new to the country, was attended with so many difficulties as to discourage the use of them.

The double mould-board Plough is very clever, and seems well calculated for the purposes it is designed for. Mr. Tugwell uses it to make the water furrows on his land. His manner of doing this on sidelong grounds, is well deserving attention. Instead of furrowing down the slopes in the usual way, he draws his furrows across, but inclining sufficiently with the declivity for the water to draw off, by which means every part of the ground is thoroughly and equally drained; and the bottoms of some of his grounds, which, in the common method, were poisoned with wet from the upper part, being now laid quite dry, are become the most productive parts of the fields.

This gentleman is likewise constructing a roller, which promises to be a very useful implement.

I saw two rollers in this neighbourhood, on a construction new to me; one of them was procured from the neighbourhood of Marlborough—a common roller, of about fourteen inches diameter, is surrounded with wheels nine inches distant from each other, and three feet in diameter; the spokes being let into the roll. The other is an improvement from this; a smaller roll is the axis, on which are put solid wheels, about three feet in diameter, and one-half inch thick; made alternately of wood and cast iron: the wooden ones are made to fix at any distance; between two of these an iron one is put one-half inch less in diameter, and with room sufficient to play up and down, so as to give way to any obstacle, and to press down into the hollows; it likewise, by these means, is rendered less liable to choak up in rough land. For breaking clods, or in light land, where great pressure is wanting, these appear to be very effective implements.

There appears to be a great deficiency of shed room in this district. Implements of husbandry of all sorts, are either left in the grounds, where last used, or at best, have only the shelter of a tree to preserve them; nor are the yards much better accommodated for wintering cattle.

This

This is a very material object; the injury sustained by having the implements thus exposed, is, perhaps, more than equal to the fair wear of them, and would well pay for the construction of sheds for their preservation. In regard to live stock, it is still worse; cattle fed on straw, in exposed and unsheltered situations, are sure to sink considerably; and are liable, when spring comes on, to the yellows, and other complaints, which greatly injure, and sometimes prove fatal to them. Dairy cows, in the open fields, down in the vale, are known to sink very much, in bad winters, though foddered with good hay. On the contrary, where good yards are constructed, with plenty of shed room, and attention is paid to littering them down occasionally, and keeping the cattle dry and comfortable, they sometimes even improve on the straw, and are sure to come out healthy and thriving in spring.

The land is chiefly in an inclosed state; but in some instances, additional partitions are wanting; the fields being too large for the proportion of the farm for any particular crop, which is attended with great inconveniencies; some open fields remain, but are fast disappearing. Inclosures have been uniformly attended with great advance of rent, and increased produce.

Population increasing. Wages and price of labour on the advance.

Draining Land, chiefly done with stone, but not sufficiently attended to.

Paring and Burning practised, and with the turnip and clover system, very much approved.

Woodlands, chiefly beech, very much decreasing and doubled in price within these twenty years. Large additional plantations are very much to be wished for, not only

only for future supply, but from a conviction founded on experience, that bleak situations, are very much improved by the shelter they afford.

Roads in general, good and improving.

The Woollen Manufactory is carried on to great extent in this district; the fine trade is at present at a stand, but the coarse for army cloathing and the East-India company remarkably brisk. The introduction of machinery, for every process the wool goes through to the loom, has thrown many hands out of employ; and several gentlemen, I have consulted, attribute the enormous rise of poors rates entirely to that cause; these, I have been credibly informed, amount, in some instances, in the immediate vicinity of the manufactories, to six shillings in the pound and upwards yearly. But I am inclined to ascribe this heavy burthen on the landed interest, more to the vicious and profligate habits of the weavers, who can, if good hands, earn a guinea and a half a week; which, supposing the carding and spinning machines to have deprived the women and children entirely of employment, is certainly sufficient, properly laid out, to maintain their families comfortably. But the misfortune is, these earnings very seldom find their way home, but are wasted in a public house, whilst the families are cloathed and fed at the expence of the parish, and the men themselves, notwithstanding their great earnings, are ragged and miserable in appearance; and in the event of a week's illness, or a temporary suspension of the particular branch of the manufactory they are bred to, are reduced to the greatest distress. This evil is not peculiar to the clothing manufactory, but is common to all I have had any acquaintance with; it is a complicated evil, and, if capable of any remedy, requires a much abler pen than mine to point out the means.

E   VALE

VALE OF BERKELEY.

For the account of this part of the county, I must beg leave to refer to Mr. Marshall, his very respectable sources of information, and the pains he has taken in describing every thing worthy of notice in the district, has put it out of my power to make any useful additions. For the same reason I leave in his hands the dairy management of the county; his account of the process in manufacturing cheese and butter, is, to the best of my knowledge, perfectly accurate and just. To his account of making butter, and to Mrs. Chevalier's letter, Annals Agri. Vol. 5, page 509, and other similar communications in that valuable publication, I would beg leave to refer, for methods infinitely preferable to the mode of churning the whole of the milk together, mentioned in some of the reports already in circulation. Cleanliness in every particular, however, is one of the chief requisites, in making sweet and good butter.

The VALE for a few Miles round GLOUCESTER.

Soil, deep and rich, varying from light sandy loams to the stiffest clays. In climate, not so forward as might be expected from the situation, owing, no doubt, to the inconveniencies the agriculture of the district at present labours under, which will be noticed in their proper places.

A vast deal of land in this district is the property of the church. The whole parish of Barnwood, a great part of Wooton and Cranham, and nearly all Tuffley, with many estates in every parish in and near the city, belong to the dean and chapter of Gloucester; the parish

of

of Maisemore to the bishop of Gloucester; and several
estates to colleges at Oxford. The church has likewise
the tithes of several parishes. The property belonging
to the colleges is now mostly sold out on lease for
twenty-one years, renewable every seven. The bishop's
land is in general sold out for three lives; when one
drops, putting a fresh one in as the parties can agree.

The Properties, with some few exceptions, are small.
The occupations are from £50. to £100. a year; some
few larger.

The Meadow and Pasture Land is in general very good,
and is employed both in dairying and grazing; but mostly
the former. The cows, the old Gloucestershire breed,
mostly reared, and very good. Oxen are chiefly of the Herefordshire and forest of Dean breeds. They are fed on grass,
hay, corn, either whole, or ground, and oil cake; the
latter, from its extravagant price, getting out of use of
late years, being advanced from four or five, to six and
seven pounds per ton.

There is very little land capable of irrigation in this
district, the brooks being extremely shallow in summer.
Large tracts of rich grass land on the banks of the rivers
Severn and Leddon, are liable to be overflowed by the
freshes, and tides, to which they owe their extraordinary
fertility. A canal from Gloucester to Hereford is now
cutting across these meadows, which shews, they were
in former times low, sour, unproductive marshes; the
soil to the depth of ten feet or upwards, being composed
of the rich particles deposited by the floods in the course
of ages. An entire wall, and several other proofs of
their original state, have been dug out, in the course of
this work. These meadows might at a moderate expence,
by the construction of proper banks, and flood gates, be
defended from mischievous floods, which sometimes

destroy

destroy the grass and hay nearly made, and receive the full benefit of those that came at seasonable times. This has, in one or two instances, where they are private property, been in some degree effected; but being, generally speaking, subject to common rights, no improvement of this kind is thought of. The following account of this description of property, in the vicinity of Gloucester, I had from very good authority.

The Town Ham, about 50 acres, common all the year round to the freemen of Gloucester for horses and cattle, and to the butchers for sheep. The butchers, old records say, have this privilege on condition of their giving the sheeps heads and plucks to the poor; but this part of the bargain is forgotten.

The Oxleaze, about 40 acres, the property of the mayor and burgesses to the 5th July; after that, common to the freemen without stint.

Portham, about 90 acres, private property to July 18th; after that, common as the Oxleaze.

The little Meadow, 60 acres, the property of the dean and chapter to July 18th; after that, common to the freemen for 3 horses or cattle each.

Mranham, 60 acres, private property to July 18th; after that, common like the little meadow.

Wallham, about 200 acres, a lot meadow, when the hay is cleared, common, without stint, to those who occupy a tenement in the neighbouring hamlets. In this meadow the lord of the manor has the privilege of turning two colts whilst the crop is growing. Mr. Marshall exclaims against this " diabolical privilege," as he
calls

calls it; but it ought, in justice to the present owner of the privilege, to be mentioned, that he offered some years ago to relinquish it on equitable terms, but the offer was refused!

Sud Meadow, about 160 acres. The land belongs to several proprietors, but a great part of it to the Duke of Norfolk. The duke has an exclusive right of common for sheep to the beginning of May; it is then trained up for mowing, and the hay being cleared, the occupiers have a right to put in two cows for each acre, and the duke horses and sheep without stint.

There is a great deal of this species of property between Gloucester and Tewkesbury, and likewise on the banks of the Severn and Avon, in the neighbourhood of that town.

ARABLE MANAGEMENT.

On the every year's land, the usual course of crops is barley, beans, wheat; or barley, clover, wheat; the clover latterly much increased, and found to answer very well.

Some of the stiffest clays are fallowed every third year, viz. fallow, wheat, beans. A great deal is fallowed every fourth year, fallow, barley, beans, wheat, which seems to be a much preferable course. On the light soils, "frouse," or peas and beans mixed, are frequently sown, and produce greater crops than either single, being a mutual support and shelter to each other.

Manures, are town dung, and that made by stall-feeding cattle, and by wintering the store cattle in the farm yards, on the barley straw, which is the only straw usually consumed on the premises. If an advance in the price of manure, is a proof of improving husbandry, this district has that proof, very decisively. A few years ago,
the

the stable dung of the largest inns might have been contracted for annually for a trifle; one of them was even threatened with an indictment, from the moisture of the accumulating dung heaps overflowing the neighbouring cellars. It is now fetched away fresh from the stable at 4*s*. or 5*s*. per waggon load.

Soaper's waste Ashes, which, in the remembrance of many, the farmers were paid for hauling away, and which could not be got rid of even in that way, are now fetched as fast as made at 2*s*. 6*d*. or 3*s*. per waggon load. These on cold, sour, grass lands, are found to be extremely beneficial.

Glue-makers Refuse, is found to be a very strong manure. On grass land it forces great crops, but cattle will not pasture on it for two or three years. It is equally efficacious on corn land; but in the instances I have known it used, it has been fresh from the yard, and without any mixture, in which cases its effects have been too forcing, running the corn up too much to straw, and causing it to lodge. If made into heaps, with yard dung and mould, and well mixed together, it would, I do not doubt, be found much more beneficial.

IMPLEMENTS.

Ploughs without wheels, long in the beam, do their work well, and perhaps, not much to be improved, at least during the present open field system. Ploughing in general done very well, and much improved of late years.

Dung Carts, mostly broad wheels, made to let up with swords.

Waggons with six and nine-inch wheels, frequent, to haul dung; no others admitted toll-free through one of the turnpikes. The waggons in general not so lithesome as on the hills.

Horses mostly used, three to five to a plough, according to the work. Some oxen, and coming more into use, which is a very desirable circumstance.

SEED PROCESS.

Wheat, is sown from the end of October to Christmas, most in November. If on clover, the clover is " brushed," ploughed light, some time before. The seed earth is given immediately before sowing, from five to eight inches deep. The land is trampled by leading horses over it before sowing, to close it, otherwise the plant is apt to perish: perhaps if sown on a stale furrow it might be better, but that is rarely practised. If sown after beans, the stubble, previous to ploughing, is rolled, harrowed, and collected in heaps and burnt. After the seed is harrowed in, the furrows are opened by the plough, shovelled out, and the land mended. It is generally rolled in spring, and twice hoed. The wheat stubble being left long is immediately mowed, and used for thatching ricks, barns, &c. the straw being sold at a great price to Gloucester. The land is brushed as soon as possible; it is again ploughed deeper the beginning of winter, and once or twice more in spring, with occasional dragging and harrowing for

Barley, which is generally sown in April, and is the crop most usually dunged for, if any. Broad clover is the only sort sown, about 10 or 12 lbs. per acre; mowed for soiling horses, and for hay; second crop mowed for hay, or seeded.

Beans.

Beans.—The land being previously ploughed, is harrowed as the weather permits, from the middle of February to the beginning of March; beans, or pouse are planted by hand across the ridges; they are twice hoed, and, if clean beans, usually reaped.

Quantity of seed sown and average produce.

seed sown.		average produce.
Wheat,	2 bushels -	20 bushels per acre.
Barley,	3 bushels -	25 bushels.
Beans,	3 bushels -	24 bushels.
Pouse,	3 bushels -	30 bushels.

Customary bushel 9¼ gallons.

The above account is of the best management in the district, in which management, I have known the bean stubbles lightly skimmed and cleaned previous to the seed ploughing for wheat; and the wheat stubbles, if foul with couch grass from awkward seasons, summer fallowed for barley. I do not think Mr. Marshall's account of the bad management and foulness of the land at all exaggerated, in many instances some years back; but, am happy to learn, that the slovenly managers are fast disappearing, and better practices daily getting ground. What Mr. M. says concerning sheep, does not respect the immediate vicinity of Gloucester, where they are never thought of for fallows, nor kept in any quantity to my knowledge. The few that are kept, are chiefly, and, from the soils being so subject to rot, ought always to be yeaning ewes, bought in after Michaelmas, and fatted with their lambs in the course of the following summer. The average produce as above stated, which I had from very respectable authority, seems very small on such rich land, but may perhaps be accounted for by the awkward

situation

situation of the arable part of the district, which is chiefly
open field, and so much intermixed, that four or five acres
is a large quantity for any man to have in a lot. I know
one acre which is divided into eight lands, and spread
over a large common field, so that a man must travel
two or three miles to visit it all. But though this is a
remarkable instance of minute division, yet, it takes
place to such a degree, as very much to impede all the
processes of husbandry. But this is not the worst ; the
lands shooting different ways, some serve as headlands
to turn on in ploughing others; and frequently when the
good manager has sown his corn, and it is come up, his
slovenly neighbour turns upon, and cuts up more for him,
than his own is worth. It likewise makes one occupier
subservient to another in cropping his land ; and in water
furrowing, one sloven may keep the water on, and poison
the lands of two or three industrious neighbours. If the
several interests in these fields could be reconciled, the
different properties laid together, and an inclosure take
place, there is no doubt, but, from the improved state
of the land, from its being laid dry and healthy, with the
introduction of a correct course of crops, more than double the quantity of corn would be raised.

Tithes, are chiefly compounded for ; arable land at 6s.
and grass land at 2s. 6d. or 3s. per acre ; but only yearly,
and therefore, in the event of an improved husbandry,
the full value of the tithe would doubtless be exacted.

Wages, in winter 12d. in summer 18d. and beer. The
harvest month about 30s. and board. Much work of all
kinds done by the piece.

> Setting beans 18d. to 20d. per bushel.
> Hoeing ditto 7s. per acre, twice over.
> Ditto wheat 5s. ditto, twice over.

F

Reaping

Reaping beans 6s. to 7s. per acre.
Ditto wheat 5s. to 5s. 6d. ditto.
Mowing, raking, and cocking wheat stubbles 20d. per
acre.

Draining, is not sufficiently attended to. Underground
drains are hardly known, nor are they wanted in many
instances; the damage proceeding more from surface
water, than from springs. The trenches and ditches
opened for this purpose, by good managers, are rendered
inefficient by the shameful neglect of the common ditches
and brooks, which not only check this first of improvements, but frequently occasion great damage by land
floods, which might be prevented if they were kept in
a proper state. The arable land is all in high ridges,
and more attention is paid than formerly to keeping the
furrows and proper trenches open to lay the lands dry;
but this is not so effectual as it ought to be, for the reasons
before given.

Paring and Burning is not practised.

Roads, are very bad, the materials on the spot being
very soft. A great deal of stone brought from Chepstow
by water, to Gloucester Quay, and sold there at 3s. 6d. per
ton, and upwards, to mend the roads to the extent of four
or five miles in some directions. They are however in
general under very bad management. A proper attention
to forming them, and to keeping the hedges low, and the
drains open, would soon make a great alteration.

Farm Houses and Offices, in general very middling, except in the article ox-stalls, which where grazing is practised, are in general very convenient.

Manufactories.

Manufactories.—The only one carried on in this district is the pin manufactory, which chiefly employs the poor in Gloucester, and a great deal round the country. Spinning is likewise brought into the neighbourhood from the clothing country.

Poor's Rates in the villages round Gloucester run from 2s. to 2s. 6d. in the pound; rather decreasing than otherwise. In Gloucester they are very much reduced, owing to a gentleman very much interested in them, having taken upon himself the direction of the workhouse, and obliged all who wanted relief to come into it.

THE VALE OF TEWKESBURY, OR WHAT IS MORE GENERALLY CALLED THE VALE OF EVESHAM.

Soil, varies from sandy loams to clay, but mostly deep and rich. In climate, this district in general is earlier than round Gloucester.

The Properties and Farms are mostly moderate.

A large proportion of this district is arable, and mostly common field, but subject to a regular course of crops.

Here, as in the neighbourhood of Gloucester, there is a considerable quantity of lot meadow, which is common after hay-making. There are likewise in several parts of the district, summer common pastures for cattle and sheep.

The Pastures are mostly employed in dairying; chiefly the North country long horned breed, mostly reared.

Oxen for grazing chiefly bought in, of the Herefordshire and North country breeds.

F 2

Sheep.

Sheep.—Though the greater part of the district under notice is very subject to the rot, insomuch that it is reckoned they lose their flocks once in three years on an average, there is a considerable quantity kept, the farmers being persuaded they could not raise corn without them. The arable fields after harvest, are stocked without stint. When spring seed time commences, they are confined to the fallow quarter of the field, and stinted, in proportion to the propervies; they are folded every night, and kept so hard, that scarce a blade of grass, or even a thistle escapes them ; and this management is thought essentially necessary, especially on the stiff soils, to keep them in good order, such soils being too hard to plough in very dry weather, and of course, not eligible in wet. The grass and weeds, without this expedient, would often get so much a-head as not to be afterwards conquered. The fold likewise is reckoned very valuable. Wether sheep are bought in for this purpose, an ordinary hardy mixed breed.

There are some inclosed parishes in this district, such as Kemerton, Bickford, and others, consisting chiefly of good sound loams, healthy sheep land, in which breeding flocks of very good sheep are kept, mostly of the Cotswold breed. In these the following are the usual courses of crops. Turnips, barley, beans, wheat, and turnips, barley, clover, wheat. In the open fields they are confined to the following course: fallow, barley, beans, wheat; the fields being allotted out for that purpose. Clover is sown sometimes in small quantity, in lieu of beans, for soiling horses, who are tied on it by the foot, the clover being first mown, and put just within their reach, by which means they eat it up clean, and pick the land over after the scythe. Vetches are likewise sown for the same purpose, to succeed the clover; this is esteemed a very good preparation for wheat. Clover is very seldom sown

in

in quantity to mow for hay, it being thought to weaken and injure the land.

The fallows are folded, or dunged, and ploughed three or four times; good managers, always give the fourth ploughing, reckoning it highly beneficial, provided it be given before Michaelmas, and the land laid thoroughly dry for the winter. In riding over some of these fields, in the course of my survey, the difference in management, was very perceivable; some of the lands, were in a state of garden culture, not a weed to be seen, and laid perfectly dry, whilst others, having received three slovenly ploughings, and no attention paid to the water furrows, were covered with filth, and poisoned with stagnant water. It is strange, that with good examples before their eyes, any persons can be so blind to their own interests.

Barley is sown in March, as soon as bean setting is finished.

Beans are all set by hand, as early as the weather permits in February, in rows twelve inches distant, used formerly to be planted lengthways of the lands, but it is now thought better to set them cross ways, being more convenient to clean, and lying better to the sun. They are twice hoed and hand weeded. Pease are not approved here, not so well admitting the hoeing and weeding as clean beans.

Wheat sowing begins towards the latter end of October, the bean stubbles are brushed soon after harvest, and again ploughed at seed time; if the stubbles are grassy, they are breast ploughed and burnt, in the best practice, if the weather permits. The clover and vetch lands, are generally ploughed some time before sowing; after the seed is harrowed in, the land is trod evenly and firmly by men, two treading a team's work. A superior manager, Mr. Stephens,

Stephens, of *Pamington*, rakes his wheat, as soon as the
land is dry enough in spring, with common wooden rakes,
raking the land two or three times in a place, so as
thoroughly to stir the surface, at the expence of two shillings per acre; it is afterwards twice hoed in the common
practice of the district; he finds this method very beneficial, and has generally superior crops to his neighbours,
who, I do not find any of them follow his example.

Manures, are those of the fold yards and stalls, likewise stable dung, coal, and soaper's waste ashes, from
Tewkesbury.

Foot Ploughs are used, long in the beam, and do their
work very well; practical farmers say, that shorter and
more compact ploughs would not work in these soils,
except the weather and state of the land was very favourable to them. Horses are chiefly used, four or five to a
plough.

Quantity of seed and average produce.

seed sown.   average produce.
Barley, 4 bushels - 20 bushels per acre.
Beans, 4 ditto   - 30 ditto.
Wheat, 3 ditto   - 24 ditto.

Wages and price of labour.

In winter 12d. to 14d. summer 18d. and beer; women
7d. or 8d. for the harvest 30s. and diet, or £3. and 1½
bushel of malt without.

The Parish of Kemerton was inclosed, and exempted from
tithe, about the year 1772, since which time the rent
is

is very much advanced, and the produce more than doubled. Population likewise very much increased.

Draining.—The observations made on this head, in the neighbourhood of Gloucester, are equally applicable here. The wet state of the land is intirely owing to the brooks and ditches not being properly scoured and opened, to carry off the surface water. An enforced attention to this, and to the cutting new drains, if wanting, all through the vale, for this necessary purpose, would be the first and grand step towards one of the greatest improvements that can be suggested.*

Paring and Burning.—I do not find that this is practised in any part of the district, except on Oxenton Hill, in the neighbourhood of Kemerton. This is a cold thin clay soil, more adapted for pasture than corn, but occasionally broken up. Mr. John Bricknell, who is represented to me as the introducer of this practice, thinks it exceedingly beneficial. He ploughs and burns for wheat ; after harvest the stubble is breast-ploughed, and left through the winter to rot ; in spring, the land is ploughed and sowed with oats, and laid down with ray grass and clovers.

Wood is scarce, the hedges and lop of trees being the chief supply. Thorns are frequently suffered to grow on the meers in the common fields, which sometimes cause disputes between the occupiers of adjoining lands, and certainly occasion more loss than profit. Odd corners would be better applied to this purpose. Dutch withy

---

* In one of the open arable fields, I observed a considerable quantity of land, which, being too wet for the plough, lay neglected and covered with rushes and trumpery, affording only a little ordinary keep to a few cattle, but which, if properly drained, would be equal in value to any part of the field.

is

is sometimes planted in boggy bottoms, and by the side of brooks to great advantage.

Roads in the neighbourhood of Tewkesbury, are mostly good and improving; in some of the deep parts of the district they are but indifferent, but exertions are making for their improvement.

Farm Houses and Offices, in the open part of the district, are in general very middling. Cows are too much foddered in the grounds in winter, which in bad weather injures both cattle and grounds materially. Some few improvements on this head have lately taken place. In the inclosed part of the district, they are much more convenient.

Leases run from eight and twelve to twenty years, and without lease, the land is held for the term of four years; in which time, according to the established course of husbandry, it is all regularly cropped.

Tithes are, in a considerable part of this district, taken in kind.

THE OVER SEVERN DISTRICT.

Near Gloucester the soil, and management similar to what has been described. But the country, generally understood by this term, consists chiefly of the red land of Herefordshire, varying, from light sandy loams to stiff clays. In climate, it is considerably forwarder than the vale round Gloucester. It is supposed, considerably more than half this district, is under permanent meadow, and pasture; the larger part of this is employed in dairying, though about Newent, and some few places, grazing is chiefly followed. Watering meadows, is not at all practised,

tised, the course of the brooks, they say, is in general too
low for this practice. Some of the low meadows are liable
to land floods, and 400 acres on the banks of the Severn,
in the tithing of Awre, are frequently flooded, though
bounded by a sea wall, at great expence to the occupiers.

Dairy Cows are partly reared, a mixture of the Gloucester and Herefordshire breeds; when bought in, the
Staffordshire and Shropshire breeds are preferred, if the
calves are designed for the butcher.

Oxen are chiefly of the Gloucestershire, Herefordshire,
and Forest of Dean breeds.

Sheep are the Ryeland breed, lately much improved in
carcass, by being crossed with Dorsetshire and black faced
Shropshire rams, which increases the weight of carcass
and wool considerably, though it deteriorates the latter in
quality, but not in proportion to the increase of weight.
It is found by experience, that, the wool of Ryeland sheep
from the neighbourhood of Ross, will, on these pastures,
get coarser and heavier, which is universally attributed to
their being kept better, and never housed.

Courses of Crops.

On the light land, barley, clover two years, peas, wheat,
when very foul, summer fallow, and lime, for turnips,
barley, clover one year, wheat. On the stiff land, fallow,
beans, wheat likewise fallow, wheat, beans, wheat, and
fallow, barley, beans, wheat. Until within these 80
years, there was no wheat grown on the light soils of this
district. One tithing of stiff land, in the neighbourhood
of Newent (Malswick liberty) still goes by the name of
the " Pudding liberty," from having cultivated wheat, at

G   a time

a time when the sandy soils were thought too light for that grain; these were chiefly appropriated to rye, and maslin; and there is still one tithing in the parish of Dymock, called the Ryeland tithing, that being in general a synonymous term for sandy land. The introduction of lime as a manure, and a better course of crops, has now, not only brought wheat into general cultivation, but produces it of a better quality than most that is brought to Gloucester market.

Manures.

Dung from the fold yards, in which the cattle are foldered in winter with straw, and from the ox-stalls.

Lime is here in very high estimation as a manure, both for arable and pasture land. In the common practice it is laid in small heaps on the arable land, to the quantity of two waggon loads per acre, if the land is very poor; if not, three loads to two acres, and spread, and ploughed in as soon as slaked. But in the neighbourhood of Newent, it is found that their best and strongest lime, which is burnt from stone on Gorsley common, requires a different management, the small heaps crusting, and not slaking properly; whereas, if put in heaps of a waggon load, or more together, it soon falls to a fine flour, digging out quite hot; this method is therefore followed in the best practice, though attended with additional trouble. It is thought equally beneficial on light and stiff soils, binding the one, and opening and ameliorating the other. This may be called a modern manure, in the district under notice. How far the repeated use of it may answer, will probably depend on a more general culture of turnips, and other vegetable crops, and the judicious intervention of dung and other mucilagenous manures. When used on pasture land, it is well mixed with soil, and is found very beneficial.

Beneficial. It is never unnecessarily exposed to the atmosphere, which is thought prejudicial..

Marl was formerly in great request, as appears by the number of old pits, but has not been in use in the memory of any person now living.

Soaper's waste Ashes, once to be had for hauling, now risen to 6*s.* a waggon load, principally used on grass land.

Oxen are much used in tillage, particularly on the sandy soils. It is thought the canal now cutting through this country, will, when compleated, be the means of reducing the number of horses, and bringing oxen into general use, by saving the road work.

Part of the district is inclosed with live hedges ; some part is still common field. I am informed from good authority, that between 300 and 400 acres of common field in the tithing of Aure, now let at about 10*s.* per acre, would if inclosed, be worth more than 25*s.* being much better adapted for pasture than tillage.. This tithing has likewise a very rich common pasture of about 100 acres, which joining other commons, and, as is generally the case, being much trespassed and encroached on, is of very little use to the proprietors, but might by inclosure be made very valuable.

The quantity of common and waste land in the district is considerable. The forest of Dean, now pretty much thinned of its timber, subject to common rights, and considerably encroached on, consists chiefly of stiff soil,. and might, if appropriated, be converted to the purposes. of agriculture with very great advantage to the nation.

Corse Lawn contains about 2000 acres, 1400 of which are situated in the parish of Corse. The proprietors are now making application for an inclosure. A paper printed.

and!

and distributed by the promoters of this application, containing some very good reasons in favour of the inclosure, will accompany this report for the inspection of the board.

Huntley Common, a considerable tract of land, now of very little use, might by inclosure, be rendered very valuable to the proprietors and the nation.

Gorsly Common contains from 300 to 400 acres of land, chiefly on a lime-stone rock, very applicable for orcharding and corn, but in its present state nearly useless.

These are the principal waste lands in the district; there are other smaller tracts: these wastes, in their present state, are not only of very little real utility, but are productive of one very great nuisance, that of the erection of cottages, by idle and dissolute people, sometimes from the neighbourhood, and sometimes strangers. The chief building materials are store poles, stolen from the neighbouring woods. These cottages are seldom or never the abode of honest industry, but serve for harbour to poachers and thieves of all descriptions. Respecting the obstacles to the inclosure of these wastes, I shall beg leave to transcribe part of a letter from a gentleman, who has favoured me with much useful intelligence in this part of my survey. " I should think the great obstacle to the
" commons, in this neighbourhood, being cultivated,
" arises from their being, in general, the property of the
" freeholders at large of each parish, any one of whom
" has a right to tear up the fences when made; and,
" whose unanimous assent it is impossible to obtain.
" Hence land that is peculiarly proper for orcharding, as
" being on a lime-stone rock, and will indeed bear ex-
" cellent corn, affords, and that with difficulty, a bare
" maintenance for a few half-starved rotten sheep, or
" diminutive cattle. The expence attending an act of
" Parliament

" Parliament is also so great, as to intimidate persons
" from applying, unless where the common is extensive,
" as is the case in Corse Lawn. Possibly, the best step
" the legislature could take, to encourage inclosures,
" would be, to have one general act, ascertaining the
" proportions according to each freeholder's separate pro-
" perty, and then leaving it to each parish, where there
" were wastes, to inclose or not ; speculative men would
" then soon buy up the smaller shares, and there would
" be ample scope for industry ; whereas now, especially
" in a litigated bill for inclosures, no man can predict the
" expence, or even success. Another reason which pre-
" vents inclosures is, that perhaps the pasture belongs to
" the freeholders, the soil to the lord ; hence arises a dif-
" ficulty in reconciling interests of so contrary a nature.
" Different commons also, are under different tenures ;
" and in some few instances such uncertainty prevails,
" that legal determinations could alone settle the point.
" Possibly too, the state of the roads may induce some
" persons to avoid inclosures ; roads over commons, have
" seldom much assistance from the surveyor, hence, per-
" haps in a wet season, fifty yards on each side the usual
" track is cut to pieces, rather than be at the trouble of
" making one good road in the middle. This is wretched
" policy, but I fear too often the case. You will re-
" collect also, that, a common is principally serviceable,
" to those only, who reside near it, and who can, there-
" fore, have an opportunity daily of seeing their stock on
" it. Persons of this class, not unfrequently throw cold
" water on every scheme to inclose, as it appears to lessen
" their own advantages, by making others joint par-
" takers with them. They forget, that ten acres, well
" cultivated, yield a larger produce than a greater num-
" ber in a state of neglect."   .

I avail myself of the same respectable authority, for an
account of the orcharding and woodlands of the district.

" It

" It is, I believe, impossible to make any accurate cal-
" culation, with respect to our quantity of orcharding in
" this district, without an actual survey. The produce
" of the inferior fruits, being used as small beer, and
" the allowance to the labourer large, not less than one
" gallon per day the year round, and two gallons a day
" in harvest ; the farmer is naturally anxious, to have
" as much orcharding as will supply him with a suf-
" ficiency, without his having recourse to the maltster ;
" he will also, supposing he has cellaring sufficient,
" always keep a reserve ; for it has been observed of late
" years, that there is not a hit, as it is provincially
" called, that is, the trees do not universally bear a good
" crop, above once in four years. Our prime fruit trees
" by no means flourish, as they formerly did ; the old
" fruits are apt to canker speedily ; and the different ex-
" periments of having grafts and stocks from Normandy,
" having totally failed, the idea has been taken up, that
" the land is tired of them, or in other words, that the
" particular pabulum necessary for the support of apple
" and pear trees, is entirely exhausted. It may be worth
" while to give Forsyth's recipe a fair trial ; and were
" this done scientifically, I should have little doubt of
" its being as successful with fruit, as with timber trees.
" Very possibly, we do not take so much pains with our
" plantations as formerly. In my own remembrance,
" wine was seldom produced, but at superior tables, and
" then only occasionally. The principal gentlemen of
" the county rivalled each other in their cyders : but
" now, the case is altered ; and cyder, and perry, are sel-
" dom introduced but at dinner, and then only for a
" draught, as small beer : after the cloth is taken away
" you must treat with foreign wines, or incur the im-
" putation of not making your friends welcome. Per-
" haps too, the method that has, I fear, too much pre-
" vailed in Devonshire, Gloucestershire, and Hereford-
                                        . " shire,

" shire, of doctoring the cyder, may have helped to have
" brought it into disrepute. Still the high prices that
" are yet given for the high flavoured cyders and perrys,
" are amply sufficient to reward the planter for his pains,
" supposing he can afford to keep it by him, till a good
" market offers. I have known Mr. Holder of *Tainton*,
" sell a hogshead of golden pippin cyder for twenty-four
" shillings per dozen, and the high prices which Tainton
" squash, and Oldfield perry, bring at the mill, are
" too well ascertained to require mentioning : unfortu-
" nately, the planter, or husbandman, is too often obliged
" to let others reap the fruit of his labours, or of a
" vintage, for want of a proper capital, or want of casks,
" and of warehouse room. As in the woollen trade, so
" in the cyder business, the factor runs away with the
" chief profit. About four or five factors, do all the
" business in this neighbourhood : they meet at Ledbury
" at an appointed day, and settle with each other, what
" they shall give ; this they uniformly adhere to, and
" the consequence is, that in a plentiful, or unplentiful
" year, the planter is little benefitted. The home con-
" sumption is small, he has no correspondence in Lon-
" don, Bristol, or any of the great markets, and must
" therefore be contented, with what the factor offers.
" Some few farmers go down to Bristol with their liquor,
" and there they meet with a fair price, far beyond
" what the factor gives, and which amply rewards them
" for their extra trouble. I suppose you are well ac-
" quainted with the fact, that the Tainton squash perry,
" is the basis of the principal part of the Champagne sold
" in the metropolis. Our trees are sometimes planted
" upon pasture, sometimes tillage ; the latter is, I be-
" lieve, the best for the trees, as it frequently stirs the
" earth about their roots, but then, great care must be
" taken not to injure the fibres. I understand, that an
" acre well planted, is looked upon as equal in value
" to

[54]

" to an acre of the best meadow. With respect to the
" soil, a sand is supposed to be the worst; a clay soil
" to produce the richest, and limestone the strongest
" cyder*. It is but seldom, that a liquor made from
" sand will last long without turning acid. Stire apple
" trees, planted at a distance from the forest of Dean,
" never make as good cyder. I had forgot to tell you,
" that our stocks are raised in a nursery, from a pro-
" miscous mixture of apple and pear seeds; that to pre-
" vent the tap root running too long, they are trans-
" planted twice, or thrice; that when they are about
" twelve or fourteen years old, they are removed to the
" place where they are finally to stand, being then worth
" about ten shillings per dozen; that in about three years
" time, they are grafted, and in about five years begin
" to be productive.

" All this district abounds with wood: there is near
" a thousand acres, in the parish of Newent: Oxenhall,
" Dymock, Hempley, Pauntley, and Bromsberrow, are,
" I imagine, in full proportion. The principal part
" is coppice, though interspersed thickly with timber
" trees, oak and elm: the oak thrives most on the clay
" soil, the elm grows almost spontaneously on the sand:
" the coppice consists chiefly of oak, and ash, though plen-
" tifully mixed with hazle, beech, sally, alder, &c. It
" is suffered to grow according to circumstances, from
" fourteen to twenty years; the prime part is devoted to
" the lath, some to hurdles, hoops, &c. and the remainder
" to cord wood, for the iron furnaces, at Powick, Lid-
" ney, and Flaxley. Cord wood is now worth 10s. 6d.
" and 11s. per cord. Bark has risen in the same pro-
" portion; and the year before last was at the highest
" price ever known: last year it fell, but still sold at

* The parish of Tainton, famous for the squash pear perry, is a stiff clay.

" 5l.

" 5l. 10s. delivered at the water side. Some of our cop-
" pices at fifteen years growth, sold in 1792 at 15l. per
" acre. The attempts to make iron with just coal char-
" red, have not succeeded: the iron is too brittle, and
" requires wood charcoal; hence the neceffity and ad-
" vantage of coppices.

Coal. " In answer to your enquiries, respecting the
" vein of coal lately discovered at Borlsdon, near Newent,
" it was seven feet thick when they left off working.
" The great obstacle to continuing the works, was, the
" want of an engine to draw off the water. The property
" in that neighbourhood, is divided into small parcels,
" coal probably is under the grounds of all the different
" proprietors thereabouts, and should any one person
" erect a fire engine, he would drain the adjacent grounds,
" as well as his own, and would of consequence, subject
" himself to be undersold. To work the pits therefore,
" to advantage, either, a company should be formed, or
" stipulations entered into by the neighbours, to make
" one common purse for the engine. We are now
" going to work the tunnel, and there is the highest
" probability, that this will lead to the discovery of new
" coal pits. In boring within a few yards of it, dif-
" ferent thin strata of coal were pierced through last
" year, in the whole, about three feet thick within the
" depth of twenty or twenty-five yards. The stone in
" the hill seems also strongly impregnated with iron
" ore."

Wages, in part of this district, have been low in money,
but in some part recompenced by an extravagant allowance in cyder, which has introduced very bad habits
amongst the labourers, and occasioned great expence, and
inconvenience to the farmer in scarce years of fruit. I
find from respectable authority, that this abuse is now

likely

likely to be rectified, and that the farmers in general, are curtailing the allowance of drink, and advancing the money price of labour. In one part of the district, the Tithing of Azure, the labourers are in part, or wholly boarded, a custom I have no where else heard off; in winter they have 12d. a day, dinner and beer; in summer 12d. and all their diet, or 18d. dinner and beer.

Draining. A little draining has been done, but it is not general; some of the low ground, and stiff arable land, suffers materially for want of proper grips, ditches, and water courses, to lay them dry.

Paring and burning, is not practised.

Roads in general, very middling, they look forward to the completion of the canal, for very great improvement of the roads, not only by easing them of much heavy carriage, but, for the supply of good mending materials, which are now, in many situations, scarce and distant.

Farm Houses and Offices, in some parts of the district, are tolerably good and convenient; in others, there is great room for improvement.

Poor's Rates, are more than doubled, in the memory of one person I enquired of, who seems clearly convinced it is more owing to vicious habits amongst the poor, than to any real neceſſity.

Tithes, in two instances, in different parts of the district where I made enquiry, are compounded for on very moderate terms.

Vermin. Rats and mice, do a great deal of mischief in this, and I suppose every other part of the kingdom.

Rat

Rat catchers, in general, are almost as great a nuisance; and it is most probable encourage, rather than lessen the number of these destructive vermin. A plain and efficacious plan for the extirpation of these destructive vermin, would be a great national benefit.

Sparrows are very much increased of late years, owing, perhaps, to favourable winters, and more to the severity of the game laws, which deters many from carrying guns, that used formerly to amuse themselves by killing these and other small birds. If the annual mischief done through the kingdom by these birds could be calculated, the amount would astonish.

I have now gone through my survey, and ventured my ideas respecting the present imperfections in the agricultural system of the county, and the proper methods to be taken for their removal. If the Board of Agriculture should think proper, to print and circulate this Report through the county, I hope the gentlemen in whose hands it is put, will make their observations, and give the necessary information concerning their respective neighbourhoods, and by that means render the account full and compleat. One district I omitted mentioning in its proper place, the Southwolds, this is represented by Marshall, and confirmed by some gentlemen I consulted, to be exactly similar in soil and management to the Cotswolds. Being very distant from it, and having no acquaintance in the district, I despaired of gaining any useful information, and therefore did not attempt it.

THE END.

www.ingramcontent.com/pod-product-compliance
Lightning Source LLC
Chambersburg PA
CBHW022036080426
42733CB00007B/857